THE HAIR LOSS SOLUTION

The Secrets to Preventing Hair Loss and Gray Hair

R.W. McGillicuddy

CONTENTS

INTRODUCTION

As long as man has walked the earth, he has been afflicted by hair loss. We see evidence of hair loss at least as far back as ancient Egypt. Hair loss is a universal phenomenon. It affects almost *everyone* at some point in their lives. Hair loss is, of course, often deemed undesirable. Hair represents vitality. It represents life. Losing it can often make a person feel weak or unattractive.

Fortunately, for every problem there is a solution. It involves what I refer to as The Hair Loss Solution and a few minor, additional steps. You might wonder why this has never been revealed before. Possibly it's because it does not require any money, it can't be patented, and it can't be turned into a pharmaceutical. Perhaps The Hair Loss Solution has been suppressed so that doctors can keep performing hair transplant surgeries and pharmaceutical companies can keep selling drugs for hair loss. Or, perhaps The Hair Loss Solution is *so simple* that it has forever been overlooked.

This book is not only written for *men* who are *cur-*

rently balding. It's written for anyone. Whether you are a man or a woman, and whether you are attempting to reverse hair loss or prevent hair loss-this book will be very helpful to you. Additionally, if you are attempting to reverse or prevent gray hair-this book will be very helpful to you as well.

At times throughout this book, I may come off as a bit forceful. That is simply because I will be trying to get you to break a very deep seated habit. We all know how hard those are to break. Hair loss can cause all sorts of psychological suffering in a person. It can cause feelings of anxiety, depression, and an overall lack of confidence. There is no worse feeling than looking in the mirror and not liking what you see. The goal of this book is to be uplifting, and to help you to reverse your hair loss so you no longer have to feel these things. Any forcefulness in this book is purposely designed to be helpful, not to be critical.

CHAPTER 1- THE AHA MOMENT

I have always felt a certain amount of skepticism towards mainstream science. I cannot help but notice a paradox. Science presents itself as absolute and all-knowing, yet this is continually shown to be false as we've seen science change throughout history. There are many things that scientists used to know for a fact, up until the point that they were proven wrong.

When I started experiencing hair loss, due to this skepticism, I was not convinced that my hair loss was caused by a gene that I inherited from my parents, or from stress. These were the two things that science was claiming were the causes of hair loss. Over time, what started out as merely skepticism gradually turned into a deep, intuitive knowing that these *were not* the causes of hair loss. I cannot explain where this certainty came from, but I was already absolutely sure that these were not the causes of hair loss- even before I knew what the actual cause was. This ignited a deep curiosity within me, and I became obsessed with figuring out what the actual cause of hair loss was. One day, I finally had a realization that provided me with the answer. I have compiled the information into this book.

Science has got us all fooled into thinking that they have everything figured out. This prevents us from opening our eyes and opening our minds, and discovering for ourselves what is actually true. Science was telling us that hair loss was caused by genetics and stress, and so nobody questioned this or thought twice about it. The world was satisfied with the explanation that science had given them, and so no one felt a need to look any further. I came up with The Hair Loss Solution simply because I was not satisfied. I continued to look further, and ultimately stumbled upon the solution. I didn't discover The Hair Loss Solution because I'm smarter than anyone else, I discovered it because I was the only one looking for it.

CHAPTER 2- THE HAIR LOSS SOLUTION

Before I get into the actual Hair Loss Solution, I would just like to say a couple things. The Hair Loss Solution may sound a bit unbelievable to you at first, simply because it is something that you've never heard before. You may feel a bit skeptical, and that is understandable. I'm not asking you to believe me, I am simply asking you to *try* it for yourself. The proof is in the pudding, as they say.

I know that hair loss feels like a race against the clock. You feel like you've got to get it sorted out before all of your hair is gone. Unfortunately, this means you don't have the luxury of being skeptical. You've got to do whatever works, and you've got to do it *now*. The Hair Loss Solution works. It has worked for me, and it has worked for many of my friends and family members. It will work for you too. Here it is:

If you're familiar with laser hair removal, and how it works, then you know it works by applying *electricity* to the area with the undesired hair. Heat is a byproduct of electricity, so the hair is essentially burned away. As long as electricity is applied to the area, the hair ceases to grow. Electricity is the key.

When I was 16 years old, I had major surgery performed on my knee and I received many months of subsequent physical therapy. One of the things the physical therapists used on my knee was what's called Electric Stimulation Therapy. Physical therapists use this machine to jumpstart a muscle that has become very atrophied. It sends an electrical current through the muscle, which automatically flexes the muscle. I would sit there, very entertained, watching the muscles in my leg contract- even though it was not me who was contracting them. Surprisingly, this is how muscles work *all* the time, even when you're not hooked up to the Electric Stimulation machine. Every time you *think* that you're flexing a muscle, what's really happening is your central nervous system is sending a current of electricity through that muscle. The electricity is doing the flexing, not you. Again, electricity is the key.

Now, if you've ever noticed, most people tend to raise their eyebrows up and down when they speak. It is a very common mannerism that we often use in order to place emphasis onto whatever it is we're saying. Perhaps, some of us do it to appear more animated or more expressive. Whatever the reason is- we all do it. Constantly. If you've never noticed this before, take a look around and it won't be long before you see someone doing it- or you catch yourself doing it.

By this point, you're probably wondering why I am rambling on about laser hair removal, Electric Stimulation therapy, and eyebrows. Well, if you put these three things together, it becomes clear that every time you raise your eyebrows you are performing laser hair removal on your own head. <u>This is *The Hair Loss Solution.*</u> To be more precise, the solution is to *stop* moving your eyebrows.

Whenever you raise your eyebrows, you are contracting the muscles in your forehead and scalp (right where your hairline is). By contracting these muscles, you are sending electricity to the area via the nervous system. This electricity is frying the hair out of your head, just like laser hair removal does.

If you were to look at a diagram of the muscles on the human skull, it would be easy to see how this would cause a receding hairline. The muscle that raises your eyebrows literally runs right along the hairline. It would also be easy to see how this would cause a balding crown on the back of the head. We have a muscle on the back of the head that sits right underneath the crown. When we contract the muscle on our forehead that raises our eyebrows, we also automatically contract the muscle on the back of the head. It's kind of like trying to bend your pinky without bending your third finger. All of the muscles in the head just have a tendency to flex together, even if you're not trying to flex all of them. Sometimes we may see a man who has a receding hairline but no bald spot, or vice versa. This is simply because the man was born with larger muscles on his forehead and smaller muscles on the back of his head, or vice versa. It's like when you see someone at the gym who has very large biceps, but a small chest. Or you see someone with big calves, and small shoulders. Everyone is born with certain muscles that grow very easily, and certain muscles that don't grow very easily. Of course, we often see men with *both* a receding hairline and a bald spot. This just means that they have developed muscles on both the front and back of the head. The last area of the head to lose hair is always the top of the head. This is because there are no muscles on the top of the head. Sometimes, we see a man whose hairline is more receded on one side of the head than on the other. This is because that man has a habit of raising the individual eyebrow on that side of the face.

We can probably get away with raising our eyebrows sometimes, *gently.* But the problem is when we do it too often and too forcefully. It's also a problem when we hold them up for too long at a time. If you are forcefully jamming your eyebrows up as high as they can go, which is what many people do, then large amounts of electricity are being delivered to the scalp. It's like having the light switch on, and the electricity is just pouring in. This is when noticeable balding appears.

There is, of course, a big difference in the way that men and women experience hair loss. Women don't experience hair loss nearly as much as men do, simply because women have smaller muscles. Men naturally have higher levels of testosterone, and so men's muscles are more developed than women's muscles. This includes the scalp muscles. The bigger the scalp muscle you have, the more hair-zapping electricity you produce when you move your eyebrows. Lack of testosterone is also the reason why children don't experience balding. Balding typically starts affecting men right around the time that their testosterone levels start to go up, and muscles start to grow.

Women may not experience hair loss in the form of a receding hairline or a bald spot, but they still experience hair loss in the form of *thinning*. Thinning hair occurs for the same reason that the other forms of hair loss occur. It's a result of moving your eyebrows too much. Women move their eyebrows up and down just as often as men do. Even though women's muscles are not as large as men's muscles, they still have muscles- so they are still doing damage to their hair when they move their eyebrows.

Typically, even in men, thinning happens first, and then the hairline starts to recede after that. If women had just a little more testosterone, it would likely be enough to push them over the edge into receding hairline territory. Fortunately for them, they don't.

You will hardly ever see a balding Native American, or a photograph of one. Native Americans have a very stoic nature, and as a result they tend to keep their faces very still. They're not raising their eyebrows very much. Different races of people actually bald at different rates because of varying levels of *pigment* in the hair and skin. The heat from the electricity of the nervous system gets absorbed directly into the pigment of the hair. We've all experienced this phenomenon when we've burned our bare feet on black asphalt on a hot, sunny day. The more pigment that something has, the more heat it absorbs. If you have dark hair, it is going to absorb more electricity than lighter colored hair. *But*, if you also have darker skin, then the skin will absorb and offset some of the electricity and help to keep the electricity away from the hair. Unfortunately for me, I have the least convenient combination of hair color and skin color as far as balding is concerned. I have very dark hair and very light skin. This means that when I raise my eyebrows, almost 100% of the electricity gets absorbed by my hair and none by my skin. This is why white people, in general, experience the most hair loss. There is no pigment in the skin to offset any of the electricity going to the hair. The most optimal combination you could have would be very light hair, and very dark skin- such as an Australian Aboriginal. Unfortunately, most of us are not of Australian Aboriginal descent. But fortunately, once you break the eyebrow-moving habit, it doesn't matter what combination of hair color and skin color you have because there will be no more electricity being delivered to the scalp.

By this point, it is obvious what you must do. You must give up your habit of compulsively raising your eyebrows. It's a matter of becoming more conscious of your facial movements when you speak, and to catch yourself whenever you're doing it. This doesn't mean that you have to become a robot or maintain a perpetual "resting bitch face." Just try to reduce your facial movements as much as you can. You'll find it's actually not that hard to speak with someone, expressively, without having to raise your eyebrows at all. But, when there is no one around, there is no reason to be contracting any of the muscles in your face or scalp. Making sure to relax all the tension out of your face while there is no one around makes it much easier to do so when someone does pop up and you need to speak with them. There's much less of a chance of raising your eyebrows if there's no existing tension lingering in the face and forehead.

People's initial fear with this concept is that if they stop moving their eyebrows while they talk, it will make them look strange or robotic. I can tell you from my own personal experience of practicing this that no one has accused me of looking robotic. I would even go so far as to say that it makes you a more easy-going person. Sometimes, people who raise their eyebrows too much give off a bit of an aggressive vibe. They can also seem like they're trying a little too hard to convince you of something. Once you break this habit of "hyper-eyebrow motion," you'll *feel* much more balanced and relaxed- and this comes across to people when you speak.

Simon Cowell, of America's Got Talent, is a very good example of someone who virtually *never* moves his eyebrows and, as a result, has no receding hairline. Guy Fieri of the Food Network is another person who moves his eyebrows very little and therefore also lacks a receding hairline. Guy Fieri is furthermore a good demonstration of how you can still appear animated and lively without having to move your eyebrows very much. I don't think anyone would describe Guy Fieri as appearing robotic. I challenge you to think of any male celebrity, and then look them up on Youtube and watch them speak. Invariably, if they are balding, they will be moving their eyebrows very much. If they are not balding, they will invariably be moving their eyebrows very little. It becomes more obvious the more you start to pay attention to it. But it is worth noting that you may occasionally see a male who moves his eyebrows a lot, but is not balding. This is due to a lack of testosterone, and muscles that are unable to grow- no matter how much you use them. Also, celebrities aren't necessarily the best examples because many of them have had hair transplant surgery.

At first it seems to be a very difficult habit to break but, in my own experience, I was able to reduce my eyebrow motion by around 90% in just three months. And then the last 10% in another month or two. Just be patient and don't try to break the entire habit in one day. Breaking the habit a little bit at a time will suffice. It is also worth noting that breaking this habit is about releasing tension from the face and *relaxing* the face. You cannot *force* your eyebrows to be still. If you try to force them you will create tension in the area, and this will have the opposite effect that you desire.

If you are really finding it difficult to break the habit, I would suggest exercising. One of the reasons why we feel an urge to move our eyebrows in the first place is because we have extra, bottled up energy. I would suggest doing 30-40 minutes of intense exercise whenever you're finding it difficult to keep your eyebrows still. You could use an exercise bike, a treadmill, or lift weights. It doesn't matter what you do. All that matters is that you workout very intensely for those 30-40 minutes. You will feel much more relaxed afterwards, and you'll find it much easier to not move your eyebrows.

The results you get from breaking this habit are

twofold. Muscles shrink the less that you use them. Every day that you go without raising your eyebrows, not only do you preserve your hair- but you shrink the muscles a little bit. Over time, the muscles will become smaller and smaller. So, on the rare occasion when you *do* raise your eyebrows, it will do far less damage to the hair than it did before. The smaller the muscle, the less electricity.

If the idea of totally halting your eyebrow movement seems too daunting for you, then you don't have to stop moving them 100%. You could reduce your eyebrow movement by 50%, and this will reduce your rate of balding by 50%. Or, you could even just reduce it by 25%. Anything is better than nothing. Of course, I recommend reducing it by 100%. Otherwise, you'll still eventually go bald- it will just take longer.

Before you try to dismiss The Hair Loss Solution as being total nonsense, let me ask you a question. Do you move your eyebrows? I already know the answer is yes because, otherwise, you wouldn't be reading this book. So, how can you be so sure that this idea is nonsense if you haven't tried to stop moving your eyebrows? You have to at least try it, before you dismiss it. Did you really think that hair loss was genetic? Did you really think the universe would doom you like that? Saying that hair loss is genetic is like saying that some trees were meant to not have leaves. When a tree loses its leaves prematurely or permanently, it's because the tree is sick-not because the tree was designed to be that way. I'm not saying you're sick, but what I am saying is that hair loss is not natural and it's not genetic. People are very quick to dismiss things as being genetic because they don't want to take responsibility for them. But, unfortunately, you can't change anything unless you first take responsibility for it.

CHAPTER 3-
DEBUNKING
OLD MYTHS

Perhaps at this point, you still have a bit of skepticism within you. Perhaps you are asking yourself, "if The Hair Loss Solution *is* true, then why is *this* guy the only person who knows about it?" Well, I have a few things to say to that.

The first thing I would say is that I don't think that I am the first person to discover this. The cure to scurvy has been discovered multiple times throughout history. It was discovered, then forgotten about, then rediscovered, then forgotten about again, etc. Its most recent discovery was in the 18th century. I think the same is likely true with The Hair Loss Solution. I think it *has* been common knowledge at certain times throughout history, and then forgotten about. Humans are a species with amnesia.

In addition, there is no money to be made from this by the pharmaceutical industry. The official narrative is that there is no cure to baldness, there are only treatments. This narrative comes to us directly from the pharmaceutical industry itself. Are you really going to believe anything that the pharmaceutical industry tells us? It is in their best interest for there not to be a cure to *anything*. Their goal is to provide us with a treatment, not a cure, that will alleviate our symptoms. We then have to take this pharmaceutical for the rest of our lives in order to keep our symptoms at bay. This is how they make lots of money. If they provided us with an actual cure, then we'd only have to pay them one time for the cure- instead of giving them money for the rest of our lives for symptom suppressors. If you *are* still feeling skeptical about The Hair Loss Solution, hopefully it isn't because you are feeling defensive of the pharmaceutical industry. They are the only ones telling us that there isn't a cure to hair loss, and so they are the only ones that The Hair Loss Solution is contradicting. Are you having trouble accepting that The Hair Loss Solution is true simply because it goes against what the pharmaceutical industry tells us?

Thirdly, the scientific community is *never* going to provide us with The Hair Loss Solution. Science is often held back by it's own arrogance. In order for the scientific community to present us with a new, innovative idea- it has to admit that it has been wrong the entire time up until now. In other words, the scientific community is not going to come out and say that moving your eyebrows is what causes hair loss because then they'd be acknowledging that it took them *all this time* to figure out something so simple. They'd rather be wrong, just as long as everyone thinks that they're right. Also, the scientific community is similar to the pharmaceutical industry in a sense. It is not in their best interest to come up with an actual solution, and especially not to come up with one very quickly. If a scientist is being paid to solve a problem, the scientist won't make much money if he or she just solves it immediately. They'll make much more money if they drag it out, and claim that they need more time to solve it. They'll receive more grants and more funding. Science has created an entire industry out of *trying* to solve a problem, rather than actually solving it. As Yoda pointed out, you either do something or you don't do something. If you are trying, then you never had any real intention of doing it in the first place.

I cannot blame the pharmaceutical industry and the scientific community without also placing some of the blame on all of us as well. One of the reasons why we don't all already know about this is because, subconsciously, we don't want to know. Many people don't want to be given a cure that requires them to change or to break a habit. People are often entrenched in their ways. They want to be given a pill so they can continue to live exactly the same way as they were living before. There will even be some people who read this book, and acknowledge The Hair Loss Solution as being true, but will make no effort to stop moving their eyebrows. They will feel that their eyebrow-movement is a significant part of their personality, and that they will look too strange without it. That is fine. I'm not here to tell anyone what to do. I'm simply here to inform you about why you are experiencing hair loss. What you choose to do with that information is up to you. But, don't let your mind trick you into thinking that The Hair Loss Solution isn't true, simply because you'd prefer it to not be true. Simply because you'd prefer a pill. You can keep waiting for the next thousand years for a magic pill without any side effects. It's never going to happen.

Like I've said earlier, the goal of this book is not to convince you of anything. The point is for you to try The Hair Loss Solution for yourself. Plus, I know that I am preaching to the choir to many of the people reading this book. The very fact that you are reading a book about hair loss means that you are already open to hearing something that you haven't heard before. Not only are you open, but you are actively seeking out something that you haven't heard before. The Hair Loss Solution probably made perfect sense to you as soon as I explained it, and you don't need any further convincing. Unfortunately, I still need to address the skeptics, and so I have debunked a few of the old theories about hair loss.

Probably the most common theory that we hear is the genetics theory. For a long time, the theory was that you inherit a "balding gene" from your father. Then there were too many exceptions to that theory, so they switched it to your mother's father. Now they claim you can inherit the gene from either one. The truth is that we *do not* inherit "balding genes" from our parents or grandparents. What we do inherit, however, are habits and mannerisms. If one or both of your parents raise their eyebrows a lot when they speak, then you are likely to pick this habit up in your early, formative years- and then carry it with you the rest of your life.

The other common, alleged, cause of balding is stress. This theory is slightly closer to the truth than the genetics theory, but it is still incorrect. Any time that I've read an article about how stress causes balding, nowhere in the article does it ever say *how* this occurs. It just says that it *does* occur. This is not very helpful to the reader who wants some practical advice on how to not lose their hair. Telling someone to "stop being stressed" is not going to help very much. We have no control over the difficulties and challenges that life throws at us, and so stress is inevitable in many situations. The only part of this theory that is true, however, is that someone with a lot of stress and tension is more likely to move their eyebrows. *But,* it is not the stress itself that is causing the hair to fall out, it's the movement of the eyebrows. I am not telling you to not be stressed. I am simply telling you to stop moving your eyebrows. You could be going through an extremely stressful time in your life, but as long as you don't move your eyebrows- you won't lose any hair. You will, however, find that once you've successfully broken the eyebrow-moving habit, you will naturally feel less stressed as a result.

The most recent, alleged, cause of balding that I've heard about is DHT. DHT is short for dihydrotestosterone, and it is a natural byproduct of regular testosterone. According to this theory, the more testosterone a man has, the more DHT he will have as a result. This DHT then makes its way to the scalp, and has a hair-killing effect. The gist of this theory is that the more testosterone you have, the more likely you are to lose your head hair. But also somehow, according to these same scientists, testosterone *increases* your body hair. This doesn't make any sense. The reality is that testosterone increases *all* of your hair. Both head and body hair. The reason why these scientists *think* that testosterone decreases your head hair is because if you already have a habit of raising your eyebrows, then an increase in testosterone will speed up the balding process (because it will make your forehead and scalp muscles even bigger, delivering more electricity to the hair). *But*, if you've successfully broken the habit of raising your eyebrows, an increase in testosterone will actually *help* your head hair to grow back for the same reasons that it helps you to grow a beard or to grow chest hair. Testosterone inherently promotes hair growth.

Lastly, I'll present you with a thought experiment, which isn't proof of anything- just something to think about. If you were losing the hair on your arms due to old age, a decrease in testosterone, or an illness- logic would tell us that the hair would uniformly and evenly thin out throughout the entire arm until all of the hair was gone. The hair would not recede from one end of the arm to the other. So why would the hair on our heads recede, if hair loss was simply genetic? The fact that head hair recedes indicates that the hair is being *bombarded* by something coming from the opposite direction of the recession. The hair is being pushed back by something. Of course, that something is electricity.

Thus far, we have discussed The Hair Loss Solution, which is simply to stop moving your eyebrows. This is going to *halt* the balding process, and if you did nothing else this would probably regrow some hair in and of itself. But, you will have a much greater chance of regrowing your hair if you make an active effort towards it. The rest of this book is geared towards the regrowth of your hair, or the reversal of your hair loss- as opposed to simply halting your hair loss.

CHAPTER 4- REGROWTH

Breaking the habit of raising your eyebrows is not only the way to halt the balding process, but is an effective way to regrow the hair as well. Simply keeping everything still in your face and scalp is your best bet at anything growing back. Hair naturally wants to grow on it's own, and the only reason why it's not growing is because you're zapping it on a daily basis with your eyebrow movement.

It is important that you be patient with the regrowth process and give it time. Many males start to experience the early stages of hair loss at around 21 or 22 years old. This means that if you are 37 years old and your hairline has receded 2 inches, then it probably took around 15 years for that to happen. So, it's possible it might take years for that hair to grow back. But do not be discouraged. As soon as you break the eyebrow-moving habit, your balding is halted in its tracks. No more hair will fall out. That part doesn't take years, it happens immediately. What more do you want? You no longer have to wake up every morning and watch 50 hairs fall out when you comb your hair. Or in the case of some people, entire clumps of hair. Even if you only see one hair grow back every six months, that is still exciting. At least it's progress in the right direction. Time is the price you pay for doing something the natural way. If you want instant results, then go get a pharmaceutical or hair transplant surgery. The nasty side effects you'll experience from those things is the price you'll pay for immediacy. Even if you would rather go down the path of pharmaceuticals and hair transplant surgery, you'll still have to stop moving your eyebrows eventually. Otherwise, you'll have to keep getting a transplant surgery every few years until you aren't able to get them anymore. And the pharmaceuticals will never put a complete halt to the balding as long as you are moving your eyebrows, they will only slow the process down. You will still eventually go totally bald, even with the surgery and the drugs- it will just take longer. You may as well stop moving your eyebrows sooner rather than later.

Maybe you'll be lucky and it won't take years to grow back. Maybe it will happen much more quickly than that. Unfortunately, I cannot guarantee the extent to which your hair will grow back, or how quickly. I am not going to sugar coat it and say that you will *definitely* regrow 100% of the hair you've lost. It depends on your age, testosterone levels and a few other factors. What I *can* guarantee is that you will not lose any more hair than you've already lost, once you successfully break the habit of moving your eyebrows. And you will, in all likelihood, at least grow some hair back.

It is also important to remember the manner in which hair regrowth occurs. In the majority of cases of hair loss, the individual's hair starts to thin first- and then the hairline eventually starts to recede or a bald spot begins to appear. In the regrowth process, it is the opposite order. Your hair will become thicker first, and then eventually, you may begin to grow new hairs along the hairline. So, just because you don't see new hairs along the hairline for a while, doesn't mean you're not growing new hairs throughout the entire scalp.

The following chapters about protein, testosterone, cholesterol, enzymes and voltage go into detail about the various ways we can promote new hair growth. Just keep in mind, while you're putting these things into practice, that the most important thing is patience. You have to give it time. Don't expect results overnight.

CHAPTER 5- PROTEIN

There are a few other things, in addition to time, that can help to facilitate the regrowth process. A large percentage of your hair consists of protein, and so increasing your ability to absorb protein will greatly help your hair growth. I recommend getting some of your protein from animal sources and some of your protein from plant sources. Animal protein is a more potent form of protein, but it lacks fiber, and so it does not carry its weight very well through the digestive tract. This causes toxins to build up over time. Plant protein is slightly less potent, but it's fiber content is very helpful in the digestive process. I would say neither one is better or worse than the other, they just have different pros and cons. Good sources of animal protein are eggs, fish, bone broth, milk, cheese and whey protein powder. Of course beef, chicken, and other types of meat have lots of protein- but there is a specific reason why I am not recommending these. It will become apparent once you read The Gray Hair Solution, which is the final chapter of this book. Good sources of plant protein are quinoa, buckwheat, chickpeas, goji berries, lentils, hemp seeds, hemp protein powder and beans. Chances are, you're already consuming enough protein, but you're probably not utilizing or absorbing all of it. There are a few changes you can make to your diet in order to help your body absorb protein more efficiently.

In order for your body to assimilate any protein that you've eaten, your body must first be able to break down the protein into individual amino acids. It doesn't matter if you eat a giant steak with 100 grams of protein in it, if you don't break the protein down into amino acids- you will not absorb any of that protein. Your body has two ways of breaking down protein: enzymes and stomach acid. Enzymes are naturally found in raw food, but they are destroyed once we cook food. For this reason, I advise including a lot of raw foods in your diet. I also advise taking an enzyme supplement if you are consuming any cooked food, and chewing your food thoroughly in order to release enzymes. I go into more detail about this in the "Enzymes" chapter.

The other way your body breaks protein down into amino acids is with stomach acid. Our stomachs need salt in order to produce stomach acid, and so you should add some pink Himalayan salt to your diet- particularly on foods that are higher in protein.

Once your body has broken down the protein into individual amino acids, it then has to build the amino acids back up again into the various proteins for hair, skin, nails, muscle, etc. Enzymes are a major part of this process as well. It would also help to add some magnesium, potassium, vitamin C, and B vitamins into your diet to aid in the process of protein synthesis. All of these nutrients help to create the energy that your body needs in order to create protein. I suggest getting these nutrients from whole food sources, but it can be diffcult to get adequate amounts of magnesium through the diet. Magnesium is one of the few minerals where I suggest taking a supplement, in addition to eating magnesium-rich foods.

In conjunction with upping your protein, increasing your testosterone is going to be very helpful in regrowing your hair because testosterone also aids in the assimilation of protein.

CHAPTER 6- TESTOSTERONE

Testosterone will actually *help* you to regrow hair. If testosterone helps you to grow chest hair or a beard, then why wouldn't it help you to grow head hair? As long as you are practicing The Hair Loss Solution, and not moving your eyebrows, testosterone will be helpful in the regrowth process.

The topic of testosterone and how to increase it naturally is a much-discussed topic, particularly in the weight-lifting world. There doesn't seem to be a definitive science on how to increase it, apart from being prescribed artificial testosterone from a doctor- which I do not recommend. Much of it is subjective or anecdotal. If you were to ask any gym-goer, they would each have a different idea on how to increase testosterone. I can really only speak from my own personal experience of lifting weights over the years.

The first thing that I noticed very quickly when I

started lifting weights was how important sleep is. If I sleep very well the night before I lift weights, I have a noticeable increase in strength- which indicates an increase in testosterone. There are a few things you can do to increase your quality of sleep. One is to stop drinking caffeine. Some people feel that they need to have at least *some* caffeine. If you are going to drink some caffeine, make sure you're done drinking it in the morning or early afternoon. Consuming it later than that can have a negative effect on your sleep. Even consuming it in the morning has a negative effect on your sleep, which is why I recommend not drinking it at all. The second thing to do is to make sure you sleep for a long enough period of time. 7-8 hours is the proper amount for most people, but many people only sleep 4-5 hours. They are only able to keep this habit up because they drink caffeine throughout the day to stay awake. If you are not able to wake up in the morning feeling rejuvenated, *without* caffeine, then you probably need to adjust some habits. Tryptophan has been known to help with sleep quality. I recommend drinking whole milk as a source of tryptophan. Many people try to avoid dairy, but as long as the milk is organic and you take an enzyme supplement with it- it is very beneficial.

Alcohol is a testosterone killer. I don't think anyone has ever drank alcohol and then woken up the next morning feeling rejuvenated. I would suggest eliminating alcohol altogether if you can. If not, then I would suggest limiting it as much as you can.

Another testosterone killer is vitamin D deficiency. Vitamin D deficiency runs rampant in many places around the world due to a lack of sunlight and our tendency to stay indoors. I started taking cod liver oil a few years ago and I felt a dramatic difference. I felt an increase in energy, I was sleeping better and I felt much stronger in the gym. These are all signs of increased testosterone. Unfortunately, many people go through life not knowing that they are deficient in vitamin D, and they suffer the consequences. The optimal way to get vitamin D is from being out in the sun, but the next best way is by consuming cod liver oil or eating fish. I do not advise taking a vitamin D supplement.

Omega 3 fatty acids are another nutrient that will help to increase your testosterone levels. The truth is that a deficiency in *any* nutrient can have a negative impact on your testosterone levels. The way to avoid a deficiency is to eat a balanced, nutrient-dense diet. But, eating a balanced diet doesn't just mean you're eating fruit, vegetables, nuts, seeds, whole grains, legumes, meat, dairy and eggs. That is part of it, but it is more important that you are aware of which nutrients are in which foods- so that you can be as efficient as possible. You've only got a certain number of calories per day, and you have to make them all count. You've really got to go down the list of all the vitamins and minerals, and then make sure you've got a food in your diet that contains each one. Right off the bat, I would recommend adding hemp seeds, seaweed and quinoa to your diet. These foods are very nutrient-dense, so you'll be covering a lot of vitamins and minerals with just these three foods alone. Seaweed is of particular significance because it's one of the few foods that contain iodine. Iodine is a mineral that many people are deficient in because very few people actually eat seaweed. Fish, eggs, avocados, and chickpeas are also nutrient-dense. You can do your own research on which foods contain which nutrients. Just be careful not to leave out any minerals or vitamins- especially the lesser known ones like boron or chromium. That can lead to a deficiency, which will in turn lead to a decrease in testosterone.

We should strive to eat as naturally and organically as possible because the toxins in our food have a negative impact on our testosterone levels. This includes staying away from fast food, fried food, refined grains, refined sugar, soda or any item at the grocery store that has a very long ingredient list. It's difficult to buy everything organic at the supermarket, but you should at least focus on the foods where you consume the outer skin of the food, like blueberries or apples.

It is best to get most of your nutrients from natural, whole foods because the nutrients are in a more bioavailable form and you also don't have to worry about taking too much. I advise staying away from supplements for the most part- apart from a few, occasional exceptions.

Lastly, but importantly, zinc is a crucial mineral in the production of testosterone. Oysters, clams and hemp seeds all contain lots of zinc.

To summarize this chapter, I would say the most effective ways to increase your testosterone would be:

- Limiting or eliminating caffeine consumption.
- Limiting or eliminating alcohol consumption.
- Limiting or eliminating processed, junk food from your diet.
- Consuming organic, nutrient-dense foods.
- Addressing any deficiencies in the diet.
- Sleeping at least 7-8 hours every night.
- Consuming more zinc.

Undoubtedly, there are other ways to increase testosterone. These are just the ones that I've seen to be effective through my own, personal experience.

CHAPTER 7- CHOLESTEROL

Cholesterol has the potential to be very helpful in the hair regrowth process. Contrary to popular belief, cholesterol, in and of itself, is actually healthy for your body. The reason why it is considered unhealthy is because we often consume it in the form of junk food, and in conjunction with unhealthy ingredients. Take a cheeseburger for instance. A cheeseburger is unhealthy, but not because it has cholesterol. It's unhealthy because it's loaded with refined salt, trans fat, preservatives, and toxins in the meat and toppings. Not to mention the lack of fiber in the white bread, and the high fructose corn syrup in the ketchup. Since we often consume cholesterol in this junk food form, "cholesterol" and "unhealthy" have become synonymous.

The reality is that cholesterol is necessary in order to create and regenerate new cells in the body. This is how a baby bird is seemingly able to be created out of nothing, in the little ball of cholesterol that we call an egg yolk. If we humans were able to float in a ball of cholesterol, it is likely that all of our hair would grow back. I say that only half jokingly because it would likely be beneficial to put some type of animal fat in your hair, like pork lard, and then wash it out in the shower. I am not saying this is necessary, but it would benefit your hair regrowth. It depends on how dedicated you are to regrowing your hair.

The best way to consume cholesterol, in my opinion, is by consuming eggs. If you can afford it, I advise buying organic and pasture raised eggs because they can otherwise contain a lot of toxins. I also recommend soft boiling the eggs so that the yolks are still somewhat runny. This maintains the potency of the cholesterol. Eggs are a superfood as far as hair is concerned because they also contain large amounts of a vitamin called biotin. Biotin is crucial in order for your body to create the protein that your hair is made of. All of the biotin in an egg is found in the yolk. Conversely, the egg white contains a protein that binds to biotin and prevents you from absorbing the biotin. For this reason, I suggest consuming only the egg yolk, and not the egg white. I recommend consuming 3 or 4 eggs per day.

The second best way to consume cholesterol, in my opinion, is by consuming fish. It's always best to go with smaller fish, in order to reduce the amount of mercury you're consuming. Personally, I think that salmon is the ideal choice because it is a fatty fish, and so it has more cholesterol than other fish. It is also very nutrient dense compared to other fish. An air fryer is a great way to cook fish because you don't have to use any oil. Just add some pink Himalayan salt or some other form of natural, unrefined salt. It is also, of course, best to make sure the fish is wild caught, if you can.

Grass fed butter is another healthy form of cholesterol. Butter does not contain lactose or casein, and so most people who have a problem with dairy should not have a problem with butter. I recommend that you buy unsalted butter because the salt found in salted butter is typically refined. You can then add your own unrefined salt after the fact. Butter is also a good source of retinol (vitamin A) which is known to be beneficial to hair.

Of course, all meats and animal products contain cholesterol, but there is a very specific reason why I am only recommending eggs, fish and butter. It has to do with these foods being very soft and easy to chew. This will make perfect sense once you read the chapter in this book about gray hair.

CHAPTER 8- ENZYMES

Although there are many components involved in the growing of hair, enzymes may possibly be the most important component. Enzymes are responsible for every process that occurs in the body. From growing fingernails to building muscle tissue to growing hair. Enzymes are also necessary for us to digest and break down food.

Unfortunately, many of us are deficient in enzymes because we eat a diet that is mostly cooked. As soon as you cook a food, you destroy the naturally occurring enzymes within the food. Your body then has to produce its own enzymes in order to digest the food. Your body is very capable of doing this, but it starts to become a huge burden for the body when 90-100% of your diet is cooked- which is actually the case for many people. If all of your enzyme production is going towards digestion, then there won't be enough enzymes to go towards other functions of the body- like hair growth.

I am not saying that you need to eat a totally raw diet, but I do recommend consuming a diet that is at least 50% uncooked. This way, much of the food you eat will basically digest itself with its own enzymes. Your body can then focus on creating enzymes for cell regeneration and protein synthesis, rather than digestion, which will result in more hair growth. Common raw foods consist of fruit, nuts, seeds, and certain vegetables. Many vegetables need to be cooked in order to be eaten, but there are a few vegetables, such as carrots or leafy greens, that do not need to be cooked. Fruit and seeds never need to be cooked, and if you're buying nuts just make sure that the package says "raw" as opposed to "roasted". Raw honey and kefir also contain enzymes. It is important to be aware that raw nuts and seeds contain a nutrient called phytic acid. Phytic acid can attach itself to certain minerals and prevent you from absorbing those minerals. This doesn't mean that you shouldn't consume nuts or seeds, it just means you should consume them by themselves- and not mixed with other foods. For instance, if you're going to eat a handful of nuts- don't eat anything else an hour before or an hour after. Hemp seeds are unique because they don't contain phytic acid, and can be mixed with anything.

There are still lots of benefits we get from cooked foods. Quinoa, fish, eggs and chickpeas are all nutrient dense, beneficial foods that need to be cooked-

and these are all foods that I recommend eating. The only point I'm making is that you should try to have a balance in the diet, so you don't end up consuming a 100% cooked diet. This way, you'll never be lagging in enzyme production, or become deficient in enzymes. Enzyme supplements are very helpful to take when we are consuming food that is cooked.

Another thing worth mentioning is that whenever you are eating food, make sure to chew slowly and thoroughly so that your body has a chance to release the enzymes necessary to digest that food. Also, the body uses many different minerals and vitamins in order to create enzymes, and so it's important to consume a diet that is nutrient dense in order to avoid any deficiencies. A deficiency in a particular mineral or vitamin can lead to your body not being able to produce certain enzymes.

Lastly, it is important to eat a diet high in fiber. Fiber is your body's main way of removing toxins. Your liver dumps toxins into fiber, and then the fiber is excreted out with the toxins. Your body also has various other ways of removing toxins, such as creating detox enzymes. The more fiber you eat, the less your body has to create detox enzymes. Your body can then focus it's enzyme production towards protein synthesis and hair growth.

As long as you're consuming lots of enzymes in your food, consuming lots of minerals and vitamins, and taking an enzyme supplement- your body will have

all the enzymes it requires in order to do everything
it needs to do, like create hair.

CHAPTER 9- VOLTAGE

Despite the fact that I have identified electricity as the main culprit behind hair loss, this does not mean that I am saying electricity is bad. On the contrary, we very much need electricity in order to function. Electricity is what allows the heart to beat, the brain to think, and the lungs to breathe. The fact that your body is animated by electricity is what sets it apart from a lifeless corpse lying on the ground. Electricity is absolutely necessary for life to exist. We could even go so far as to say that electricity *is* life. Being that hair is a sign of life, we want more electricity in the body.

The reason why electricity is causing your hair loss is because your electricity is out of balance. You have a leakage of electricity, leaking directly into your hair. We simply have to fix the leakage, which we do by ceasing to move the eyebrows. As long as the leakage is fixed and we've broken the eyebrow-moving habit, it is beneficial to increase the overall electricity in the body. Kind of like raising our voltage, so to speak. It is what traditional Chinese medicine refers to as *Qi*, and what the Hindus refer to as *prana*. In the West, it is known as *life-force*. The more we raise our voltage, the more energy we have and the more the body is able to regenerate and repair itself. This ultimately results in hair growth. The main reason why the body is not able to function, as it should, is because of a lack of energy.

We can go about raising our voltage in a few different ways. One way is to increase the health and strength of our nerves. The nervous system is the generator of electricity in the body, and so if the nerves aren't healthy- you will have low voltage. The B vitamins, particularly B12, have been known to be beneficial to nerves, and to increase overall nerve health. Clams are an incredibly good source of vitamin B12. Salmon, eggs and dairy are also good sources of B12. Nutritional yeast is an excellent way to get the rest of the B vitamins, apart from B12. Whole grains are another great source of B vitamins. Like dairy, as long as you consume *organic* whole grains and you consume them with an enzyme supplement- you should not have trouble digesting them.

The second way to raise our voltage is with electrolytes. Electrolytes are called electrolytes for a reason- because they conduct electricity throughout the body. The five main electrolytes are: sodium, potassium, magnesium, calcium and phosphate. It's important to consume these five minerals everyday because they very easily get sweated and urinated out.

Finally, consuming copper is an effective way to raise voltage in the body. Copper is a highly conductive mineral, and therefore it helps the body to produce electricity. It is very important to consume copper in its natural food form because copper supplements don't absorb very well. Oysters and clams are great sources of copper. Salmon, avocados, chickpeas and hemp seeds are some more good sources of copper. Copper also serves another purpose that is helpful to hair, which I will talk about later on in the chapter about gray hair.

CHAPTER 10- BLOOD FLOW

In the previous chapters about protein, testosterone, cholesterol, enzymes and voltage- we've talked about consuming various nutrients that will help to rebuild the hair. This is a crucial aspect of the regrowth process, but it doesn't matter how many nutrients you consume if the nutrients don't get delivered to the hair. Optimal blood flow is just as crucial as the consuming of the nutrients. Immediately after you eat food, the nutrients from the food go into your bloodstream. The blood then delivers the nutrients to the various parts of the body. If your blood is stagnant, and not flowing very well- then these nutrients won't make it to their destination. The scalp is the most difficult place for the body to send blood because the body has to fight against gravity. There are various ways in which we can increase blood flow.

Increasing the amount of iron in your diet will

help to improve blood flow. Iron is integral to the blood, and so blood without iron doesn't function very well. Iron is one of those minerals where it is very important that you get it from food and *not* from a supplement. Iron from supplements has been known to get stuck in areas of the body where it shouldn't be, and it can be toxic. Hemp seeds are a great source of natural iron. Oysters, mussels and salmon are also good sources. Sea moss is another iron-rich food that I consume on a regular basis, and it contains many other beneficial minerals as well. Vitamin C has been known to help with the absorption of iron, and so I try to eat an orange everyday- as well as taking whole food vitamin C supplements such as acerola cherry powder. I do not recommend taking ascorbic acid supplements. The whole food form is always better.

Exercise is a great way to increase blood flow. I am not going to recommend any form of exercise in particular. The only thing that matters is that it is a form of exercise that you enjoy. That way, you will be able to do it consistently without it feeling like a chore. It could be something as simple as walking outside everyday.

Getting your head beneath your heart is an effective way to increase blood flow to the scalp. You don't have to be entirely upside down- in fact, I advise not doing so because that creates too much pressure in the head. You can just lie on a bed and let your head hang off the side of the bed. You can alternate between lying on your stomach and lying on your back, to ensure the blood gets to the entire scalp. You only need to do this for a couple of minutes everyday. I have found this exercise to be very helpful.

Lastly, massaging the scalp can be very helpful in stimulating blood flow. Again, you don't need to spend a lot of time doing this. A couple of minutes everyday is enough. Just don't massage so hard that you are pulling your hair out. I would suggest massaging the entire scalp- not just the areas of the scalp with hair loss. There are various massage tools designed for the scalp that you can purchase online, and they are inexpensive.

CHAPTER 11- MAINTENANCE

At this point, we've just about covered everything. Everything from the reason why you are balding, to how to regrow the hair that you've already lost. There are a few final things that are worth mentioning. Things that are perhaps not the most crucial pieces of the puzzle, but are still helpful nonetheless.

If you have any extra money lying around, I would say it's worth investing in a water filter for your shower head. There is typically a substantial amount of chlorine (amongst other things) in tap/shower water. If you've ever known someone who was on the swim team, then you probably already know that chlorine is very damaging to hair.

The manner in which you shampoo your hair is a pretty significant factor in the overall health of your hair. There are two different ways you can approach shampooing your hair. First, it is important to note the relationship between *oil* and electricity.

Essentially, oil *cools down* electricity when electricity passes through it. This means that having more oil in your hair has a protective effect against the electricity that you create by contracting your scalp muscles. For this reason, you may not want to shampoo your hair everyday because shampoo removes the naturally occurring oils in your hair. You could try shampooing your hair every other day, or even every third day, in order to maintain a certain amount of oil in your hair. Personally, I don't follow this approach. I follow the other approach. Since I don't move my eyebrows at all, I don't need to worry about having extra protection against electricity because there is no electricity. I shampoo my hair everyday because, although oil is protective against electricity, it can also be an impediment to optimum hair growth. Oil, dirt, and sweat can all act as impediments so it is important to remove these things and to keep the scalp clear. I would suggest the first approach if you are still in the process of breaking the eyebrow-moving habit, and the second approach once you've totally broken the habit.

While showering, many people make the water too hot. This can be very damaging to the hair. I use lukewarm water while showering, or sometimes just slightly warmer than lukewarm. This can take a little getting used to, but once you do get used to it, you'll look back and wonder why you ever took such hot showers.

Immediately after getting out of the shower, the

first thing we typically do is throw a towel over our head and violently dry our hair. There is no need to do this. All it does is unnecessarily pull out hair. All you need to do is place the towel on your head and pat down. No side to side movement is necessary. Also, try to avoid blow drying your hair. Any form of heat is damaging to the hair.

Following the drying of the hair, the next thing we typically do is comb our hair. Again, most of us are unnecessarily violent with our combing. Combing too hard pulls out the hair. You should comb slowly, and gently. The same applies to using a hair brush.

If you're ever outside in the sun for an extended period of time, such as being at the beach or golfing, I would advise wearing a hat. That amount of sunlight can be damaging to the hair. But apart from these specific instances, I advise not wearing a hat. Wearing a hat can cause a buildup of sweat, dirt and oil which are not conducive to optimum hair growth.

It goes without saying that it's very important to drink lots of water and stay hydrated. I recommend drinking *natural spring* water, and finding a brand that says "bottled at the source" or "untouched by man" on the label. I recommend staying away from highly purified water. The reason I say this is because when you remove everything from water, the water is then in a very unsaturated state. It's almost like a dried out sponge just waiting to soak up anything it comes in contact with. So when you drink the water, it's going to absorb lots of minerals from your body and then you're going to urinate them out. Natural spring water is saturated and so it is already filled with minerals. So when you drink it, it's not going to take any of your minerals. Having said that, purified water is still far superior to tap water. If your only option is tap water or purified water, definitely go with the purified water.

In conjunction with drinking lots of water, it is important to not drink too much caffeine or alcohol- since these things dehydrate you. It is also important to consume lots of electrolytes (potassium, sodium, calcium, magnesium, phosphate) in order to stay hydrated. It is not necessary to drink a huge amount of water in order to stay hydrated. In fact, drinking *too much* water can actually dehydrate you because you urinate out your electrolytes. You're better off just drinking a moderate amount of water, and consuming lots of electrolytes. Coconut water and whole milk are good because they both contain many electrolytes.

A small, but notable, percentage of hair consists of lipids, or fats. If you're eating eggs, salmon and butter on a regular basis- you'll be supporting your hair with very healthy fats. Some other healthy sources of fat include avocados, walnuts and hemp seeds.

CHAPTER 12- THE GRAY HAIR SOLUTION

Fortunately for all of us, simply by implementing The Hair Loss Solution in our lives, we are automatically implementing *The Gray Hair Solution* as well. This is because it's the same principle. We've already explained how the electricity from your nervous system goes to your hair and zaps it out of your head. We've also discussed how the more pigment you have in your hair, the more the electricity is attracted to your hair because the pigment absorbs the electricity. If a lot of electricity goes to a particular strand of hair, the strand of hair will likely fall out before it has a chance to lose its pigment. *But,* if lesser amounts of electricity are going to that strand of hair, the strand itself still has a chance of surviving but the pigment will get zapped from the electricity. This is when gray hair occurs. So, just to reiterate- large amounts of electricity will cause hair *loss*, while small amounts of electricity will cause *gray* hair.

As long as we are alive, our bodies are constantly regenerating themselves. They say every seven years we have an entirely new body. This means that our bodies are continually creating new pigment for our hair. The problem is that we are continually zapping the pigment by contracting the muscles on our head. If we are zapping more pigment than we are creating, then this is when a significant amount of gray hair occurs. There are two possible solutions to this problem. We can either zap less pigment or we can create more pigment. Or, we can maximize our results by doing both. Simply by following the suggestions found in the chapters about protein, testosterone, cholesterol, enzymes and voltage- you will be helping your body to create more pigment. In addition, simply by following The Hair Loss Solution, which is to stop moving your eyebrows, you will be zapping less pigment.

There is one additional thing to take note of that applies to The Gray Hair Solution but does not apply to The Hair Loss Solution. Gray hair is not only caused by the movement of your eyebrows, but also from chewing food. If you look at someone while they're chewing food, you can see the muscles expanding and contracting over the ears and up towards the front of the head where the temples are. Oftentimes, particularly in men, this is *precisely* where you will first start to see gray hair. These might be very small contractions, and they're probably not enough to cause hair *loss,* but they are still enough to cause gray hair.

The solution to this is to simply chew your food more slowly and more gently, so you don't have to contract these muscles as forcefully. This will likely require you to designate more time for eating. The more quickly you try to eat, the more forcefully you are going to chew. Also, you may want to limit the amount of meat that you consume because meat is a particularly chewy food, especially steak. It requires extra contraction in those muscles. If you are going to consume meat, fish is the best option because it's the least chewy. Another helpful thing would be to add more smoothies to your diet, or other soft foods which don't require much chewing. If you chew gum, I suggest never chewing it ever again. Chewing gum serves no purpose other than to cause your hair to turn gray.

Earlier in the book we spoke about enzymes, and how the body requires certain minerals and vitamins in order to create enzymes. There happens to be a particular enzyme that produces pigment for the skin and hair, and the body requires *copper* in order to create this enzyme. If you have a copper deficiency, then your body cannot produce this enzyme- and your hair will eventually turn gray. It is important to have a large amount of copper (from food, not from supplements) in the diet in order to prevent this from happening. As I mentioned earlier, oysters and clams are good sources of copper.

One last factor to consider with gray hair is hydrogen peroxide. Hydrogen peroxide has been used to bleach people's hair blonde because it has a pigment-killing effect. Hydrogen peroxide is actually produced by our bodies in order to perform certain functions, but the body is supposed to be able to create enzymes to turn the hydrogen peroxide back into water. Unfortunately as we age, we create less and less of these enzymes- leading to a buildup of hydrogen peroxide and an increase in gray hair. In order to combat this problem, we simply need to provide our bodies with the minerals that are necessary in order to create the enzymes that breakdown hydrogen peroxide. There are two enzymes that breakdown hydrogen peroxide. One of these enzymes requires selenium in order to function, and the other enzyme requires manganese and iron. Brazil nuts are an excellent source of selenium, mussels are an excellent source of manganese and hemp seeds are an excellent source of iron. It is important to get these minerals from food and not from supplements.

Just like in The Hair Loss Solution, I cannot make any guarantees about how much gray hair you'll be able to *reverse*. This depends on various factors- mainly your age. I can only say that any *future* graying will be significantly reduced, if you significantly reduce the amount of chewing in your diet and you significantly reduce your eyebrow movement- and if you increase the amount of copper in your diet.

I am not going to tell you to eat an all smoothie diet because that is not realistic or appropriate for everyone- but if you are really serious about reversing your gray hair, then that would be the way to go.

AFTERWORD

So there you have it. The complete guide on how to put an end to your hair loss. And, it is 100% natural. Of course, if I didn't say it enough already, the main point in this book is to stop moving your f*****g eyebrows. Nothing else in this book will be very helpful if you don't first conquer your eyebrow-moving habit. But, once you *do* conquer the habit, everything in this book will be very helpful and effective.

I also realize that some of the suggestions I've made throughout this book can, at times, be expensive. Like I've said, the main point is that you stop moving your eyebrows (which is free), and that alone will take you a long way. Anything after that is a bonus. If you have any extra money to buy the food or supplements that I've recommended, then that's great. If you can't afford them, it's no big deal. You can still reverse your hair loss.

I hope that you don't extrapolate from The Hair Loss Solution that numbing your face with injections would be a good idea to help keep your eyebrows still. These injections are very toxic, and unnatural. Every suggestion I've made in this book is not only geared towards reversing your hair loss, but is also geared towards improving your overall health and well-being. Therefore, I would *never* promote injecting a toxic chemical into your face.

Perhaps you are someone who has not yet experienced any hair loss. Maybe someone recommended this book to you because they've seen that you move your eyebrows a lot, and they know it's only a matter of time before you start losing your hair. You are very lucky because you can simply break your eyebrow-moving habit *now*, with the confidence that you'll never go bald in the future. Up until now, men have gone through life like Russian roulette, never knowing which day will be the day that their hair starts falling out. With The Hair Loss Solution, you no longer have to leave it up to chance.

www.ingramcontent.com/pod-product-compliance
Lightning Source LLC
Chambersburg PA
CBHW051231250726
48655CB00006B/2719